LIVING THE GREEN LIFE

A Comprehensive Guide

To Embracing

Vegetarianism

KARRY WILSON

TABLE OF CONTENTS

INTRODUCTION

Transitioning from a meat-based diet to a vegetarian one may seem like a daunting task, especially if you've been consuming meat your entire life. You might question why you should even consider making such a significant change. After all, if you've been following a certain eating pattern for years, it's natural to wonder if it's worth switching now.

However, there are numerous compelling reasons why you might choose to adopt a vegetarian diet. Take a moment to reflect on your current state of well-being. Look at yourself in the mirror and ask some important questions:

Are you at a healthy weight?

Do you feel consistently good and energized?

Do you wake up each day feeling refreshed or fatigued?

How would you rate your overall health?

Are your blood pressure, cholesterol, and blood sugar levels within a healthy range?

If you find yourself answering "no" to most of these questions, it's crucial to evaluate your daily food choices. If you notice that you often feel worse after eating, you might be wondering why food has such a negative impact on your well-being.

The truth is, food should nourish and revitalize your body, leaving you feeling refreshed and energized. Your body functions like a well-oiled machine, and it requires quality fuel to perform optimally.

Unfortunately, the majority of people today struggle with weight issues, often stemming from excessive meat consumption and a high intake of unhealthy fats. This unhealthy diet leads to problems such as high blood sugar, Type II diabetes, elevated cholesterol levels, and various other health-related complications.

The good news is that all of these issues can be prevented, and even reversed, through dietary changes. This eBook aims to guide you on the journey toward a vegetarian lifestyle and demonstrates the incredible transformation you can achieve in a relatively short period of time.

By embracing vegetarianism, you will discover a wealth of benefits that extend far beyond mere weight loss. Improved overall health, increased energy levels, and a reduced risk of chronic diseases are just a few of the rewards that await you.

This comprehensive guide will provide you with practical tips, delicious recipes, and invaluable knowledge to help you make a seamless transition to a vegetarian diet.

Now is the time to embark on this exciting new chapter and unlock the remarkable benefits that await you. Let's delve into the world of vegetarianism together and uncover the incredible potential it holds for your health and well-being.

I

Embracing a Plant-Powered Lifestyle

Unveiling the Path to a Healthier You

Embarking on the journey to vegetarianism may appear challenging, especially if you have been a lifelong consumer of meat. You might question the reasons behind such a drastic shift and wonder if it is truly worth considering.

However, the world of vegetarianism is vast and accommodating, offering various options to suit your preferences and needs. Let's explore the different types of vegetarians and discover the ideal path for you:

Lacto Vegetarians: This group excludes animal products and eggs from their diet but includes dairy products like milk, cheese, and yogurt.

Ovo-Vegetarians: This category eliminates animal products and dairy but includes eggs as part of their dietary choices.

Lacto-Ovo Vegetarians: These individuals abstain from consuming any animal products while still incorporating dairy and eggs into their meals.

Vegans: Vegans adopt a plant-based diet, excluding all animal products, including dairy, eggs, meat, and even honey.

If you're uncertain about which type of vegetarianism suits you best, don't worry. It takes time and experimentation with different recipes to determine what works for your taste buds and nutritional needs.

Some individuals find it challenging to completely let go of certain foods, like milk and eggs, and that's perfectly fine.

You Truly Are What You Eat

We've often heard the phrase "you are what you eat" tossed around in advertisements, but let's take a moment to reflect on its profound meaning. Imagine gazing into a mirror that reveals not just your external appearance, but the impact of your dietary choices on your body.

Consider the example of your blood plasma. Under normal circumstances, it appears as a clear liquid. However, after consuming a high-fat fast-food hamburger, your blood plasma becomes clouded with fat and cholesterol. This vividly illustrates how the food you consume affects your body.

Conversely, when you transition from a meat-centric diet to a plant-based one, remarkable changes occur. Excess fat diminishes, and your risk of various cancers and diseases decreases.

Cholesterol levels can improve, blood pressure stabilizes, and overall health and fitness problems often fade away. Additionally, the incidence of Type II diabetes significantly reduces. Not only will you notice positive physical transformations, but you may also find yourself relying less on medications.

For individuals with a family history of high cholesterol or blood pressure, your dietary choices become even more critical. The path you choose to nourish your body directly influences your well-being.

By embracing a vegetarian diet, you can lower the risk of numerous diseases, and statistically, vegetarians tend to enjoy better health outcomes.

Uncovering Our Ancestral Diet

Have you ever wondered what our ancestors consumed and how far we've strayed from their eating habits? Originally, our ancestors were hunter-gatherers who relied on natural vegetation for sustenance. They did not consume animals as part of their diet.

A quick glance at predators and carnivorous animals reveals their sharp teeth, designed for ripping and tearing flesh. In contrast, herbivores possess flat teeth ideal for chewing plant-based foods.

Humans, too, evolved from creatures that followed a vegetarian diet. Our digestive systems were not initially designed to process and digest meat. The consumption of meat emerged as a necessity when our ancestors faced scarcity of their natural plant-based food sources. They likely believed that incorporating meat into their diet would provide sustenance.

Originally, our ancestors closely resembled herbivorous apes, walking upright on their hind limbs while foraging for roots, berries, fruits, and nuts. They lived in the present moment, constantly searching for food to survive.

Hunting required intellectual prowess, and consuming meat necessitated the use of fire. Until the discovery of fire, our ancestors primarily relied on vegetables, fruits, nuts, and berries for sustenance. Vegetarianism, therefore, aligns with our natural eating habits and promotes overall well-being.

The Shift Towards Meat Consumption

In frozen regions, where survival was challenging, prehistoric humans resorted to eating anything available to sustain themselves. Meat became a vital source of sustenance, marking a significant change in their eating habits and overall health.

Initially, the consumption of meat involved natural forest fires that provided cooked meat. In the absence of fire, raw meat might have been consumed, although the human digestive system likely faced challenges with raw meat. Over time, as humans adapted, meat became a regular part of their diet.

Some individuals who have followed a vegetarian lifestyle for extended periods of time may experience discomfort or illness if they reintroduce meat into their diet. This mirrors the challenges our prehistoric counterparts would have faced. Biologists affirm that our bodies are not inherently designed to digest meat, but rather, we have adapted to it over time.

An Ever-Present Ritual

As human civilization progressed, the consumption of meat became more prevalent. Families began including meat as a central element of their meals, leading to the development of long-standing culinary traditions.

Turkeys became the centerpiece of Thanksgiving dinners, while pork and sauerkraut became synonymous with New Year's celebrations. Easter meals often feature ham, and the tantalizing aroma of barbecues fills the air during summer gatherings.

Considering the sheer amount of meat consumed throughout history, it is remarkable to reflect on the fact that our bodies were originally designed to thrive on vegetables, fruits, nuts, and berries.

Embracing the Power of Change

When our ancestors relied on meat for survival, it was a communal endeavor. Hunting large animals like buffalos required the collective effort of several individuals. The shared labor involved in cleaning, cooking, and preserving meat created a sense of unity and reward.

Today, while we no longer need to hunt for our food, the tradition of communal meals persists. Gathering around a ham, for example, taps into thousands of years of ingrained tradition.

Food, in all its forms, remains at the heart of our celebrations. However, envision the possibilities and the transformative impact on our health if we were to transition away from meat-centric diets. Imagine the incredible variety of nutrient-rich plant-based meals awaiting our exploration.

If you recognize that embracing a healthier lifestyle could significantly enhance your well-being, then that alone should serve as a compelling reason to make a change. You need not make an abrupt transition.

Some individuals may still enjoy a refreshing glass of milk, appreciating its calcium and vitamin D content. If giving up meat entirely feels overwhelming, consider making it a side dish and increasing your consumption of wholesome vegetables. The difference in how you feel will astound you.

In the following chapters, we will delve deeper into the world of vegetarianism, guiding you through a myriad of delicious recipes, providing practical tips for success, and empowering you with knowledge to embark on this transformative journey. Get ready to experience a new level of health and well-being as you embrace the wonders of a vegetarian lifestyle.

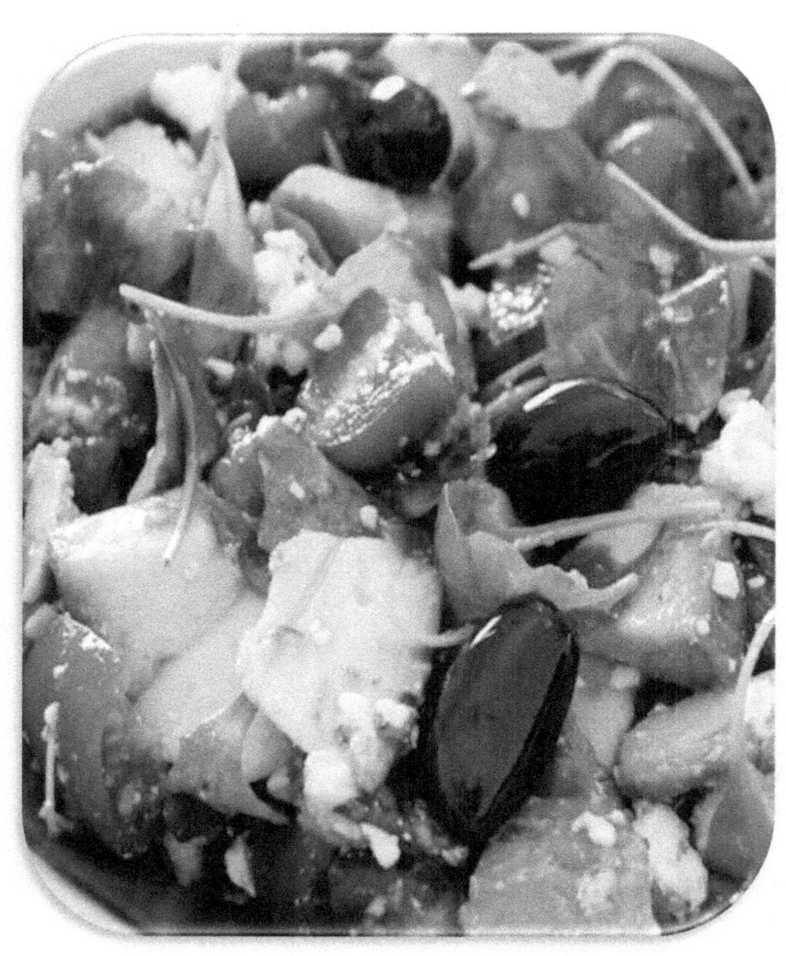

II

Understanding the Ethical Connection

For many individuals, adopting a vegetarian lifestyle is not only a choice based on health considerations but also a moral commitment to animal welfare.

Throughout centuries of domestication, humans have often regarded themselves as superior to animals, exploiting them for various purposes beyond just food, such as clothing, footwear, and scientific experimentation.

However, the perspective is shifting, and organizations like People for the Ethical Treatment of Animals (PETA) are working tirelessly to transform societal attitudes towards animals.

Unveiling PETA's Mission

PETA, an acronym for People for the Ethical Treatment of Animals, is an organization dedicated to revolutionizing people's perception of animals. PETA staunchly opposes the use of animals for any purpose, be it food or clothing, and vehemently condemns practices like fur trapping.

While their passion may sometimes appear extreme, their cause is rooted in the belief that animals possess rights and deserve consideration for their well-being.

They strive to enlighten society about animal suffering and advocate for animals' right to lead their lives in their natural habitats. PETA urges us to reevaluate our place on this planet and our relationship with its diverse animal inhabitants.

Growth Hormones and Unethical Practices

The quest to produce animals at an accelerated rate to meet human consumption demands has led to the widespread use of growth hormones in livestock. However, this raises critical questions about the treatment and conditions of these animals.

To comprehend the magnitude of the issue, consider the plight of egg-laying chickens. These birds are often crammed into tiny cages, with each chicken allocated a mere 67 square inches of space. Additionally, they are commonly subjected to growth hormones and antibiotics to enhance growth and minimize disease.

While free-range and certified organic chickens may experience more spacious living conditions and remain free from hormones and antibiotics, the hygiene precautions required when handling chicken are notable.

Bleach is recommended for cleaning surfaces to eliminate bacteria, and specific temperature and cooking durations are necessary to prevent foodborne illnesses. The need for such meticulous care raises concerns about the overall safety and suitability of consuming chicken.

Expanding our perspective to the treatment of cattle, we encounter dairy farming practices. Dairy cows are often administered hormones to stimulate their reproductive processes and ensure continuous milk production.

These cows endure cramped living conditions, and once they give birth, male calves are promptly sent for veal production while females are raised for milk.

The administered hormones cause cows to produce milk quantities far beyond natural capacity. Additionally, the use of electric pumps for milking can irritate the cows' udders, leading to discomfort.

Considering that we do not require milk beyond a certain age and that our bodies are not designed to digest cow's milk, opting for alternatives becomes a rational choice. Green, leafy vegetables provide abundant calcium and offer a viable alternative.

An Unsettling Reality

The veal industry has long faced criticism from both meat consumers and vegetarians alike due to its inherent cruelty.

Calves are separated from their mothers shortly after birth and confined to pens that restrict movement, ensuring their muscle tissue remains tender.

These calves are then fed a liquid diet deficient in iron and fiber, resulting in anemia and the production of pale meat. By approximately 20 weeks of age, these calves are ultimately slaughtered, underscoring the disturbing nature of this industry.

A Dark Tale of Confinement

Turkeys, commonly consumed not only during holiday festivities but throughout the year, are subjected to inhumane treatment as well. Due to their aggressive behavior, turkeys are kept in confined, dimly lit spaces to discourage their natural instincts.

Overfeeding is practiced to ensure larger turkey breasts, fulfilling the desires of consumers. Naturally, turkeys can live up to 10 years, yet those bred for consumption are slaughtered at just two years old.

They suffer from foot and leg deformities, heat stress, and starvation, with approximately 2.7 million turkeys dying annually due to the abnormal stress and disease inflicted upon them.

Examining the Pork Industry

Pigs, often associated with unsanitary conditions, also endure significant challenges. Methane gas produced by the vast amounts of waste in pig farms has led to the deaths of farmers and workers due to inhalation. Pigs are confined, overfed, and raised in cramped crates, limiting their natural behaviors and range of movement.

Growth hormones and antibiotics are commonly administered to enhance production. The captivity in which they exist contradicts their innate rooting behaviors, preventing them from living in alignment with their natural instincts.

Health Benefits and Mercury Concerns

While seafood and shellfish contribute to a nutrient-rich diet, offering high-quality protein, essential nutrients, and omega-3 fatty acids with low saturated fat, there are associated risks.

Fish often contain mercury, which, while generally not harmful in significant quantities, warrants caution. The Food and Drug Administration (FDA) and the Environmental Protection Agency (EPA) advise specific groups, such as pregnant women and young children, to avoid certain types of fish and shellfish due to elevated mercury levels.

The decision to eliminate fish from one's diet often marks the final step in transitioning towards a complete vegetarian lifestyle.

By considering the ethical implications of our food choices and embracing a vegetarian diet, we can actively contribute to the welfare of animals and foster a more compassionate society.

Let us venture further into the world of vegetarianism, exploring its myriad benefits and unraveling the secrets to

creating delectable, plant-based meals that nourish our
bodies, minds, and the world around us.

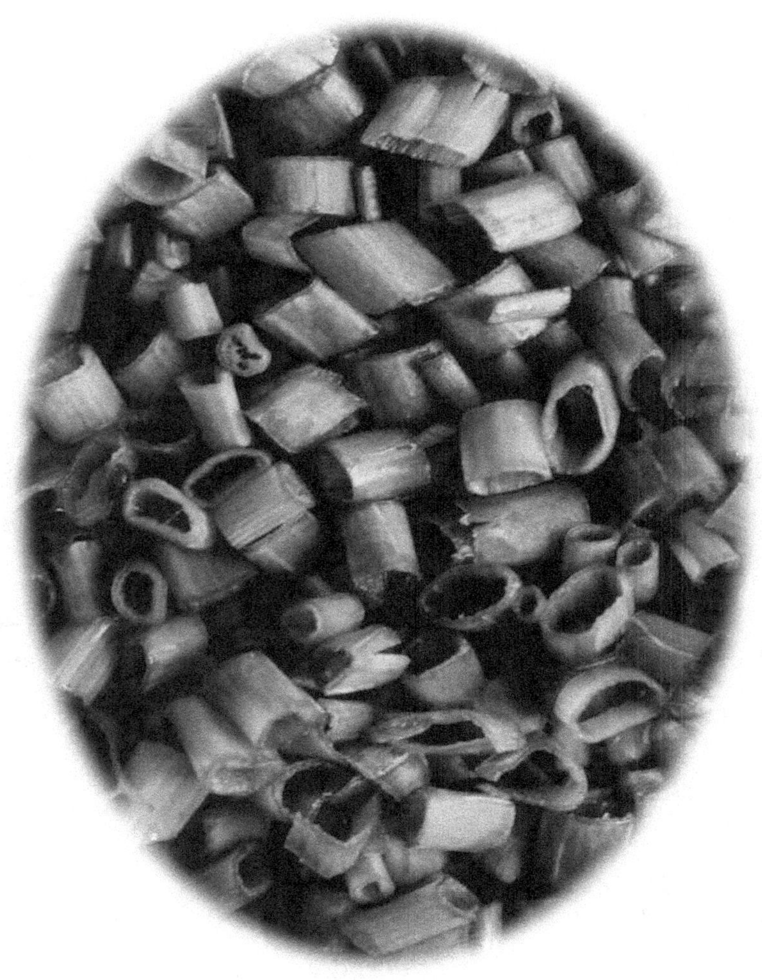

III

Thriving on Vegetarianism:
Unleashing the Health Benefits

Revelations of Vitality

Prepare to be astounded by the remarkable transformation you'll experience when you embark on a vegetarian journey. It's as if your body instantly begins to cleanse itself of accumulated toxins, leaving you feeling invigorated and experiencing a newfound sense of overall well-being.

Regardless of your initial motivations for embracing a vegetarian diet, the health benefits will become evident within a remarkably short period.

Unveiling Cardiovascular Advantages

Vegetarians enjoy lower levels of blood fats, cholesterol, and triglycerides compared to meat eaters of similar age and status. Even among vegetarians who consume eggs and milk, cholesterol levels remain lower than their meat-consuming counterparts.

Let's delve into the topic of heart disease—a leading cause of mortality. Research reveals that men who consume meat six or more times per week are twice as likely to develop heart disease.

Middle-aged men, in particular, face a higher risk of fatal heart attacks. However, older women who follow a vegetarian lifestyle exhibit a lower risk of heart disease.

A study conducted in 1982 involving over 10,000 individuals, both vegetarians and meat eaters, demonstrated a direct correlation between meat consumption and heart attack risk.

By eliminating meat from your diet, you simultaneously reduce your intake of harmful fats and cholesterol that can jeopardize heart health. It is crucial, however, to moderate your consumption of cream cheese, ice cream, hard cheese, and eggs to fully reap the benefits of vegetarianism. Embracing a diet rich in vegetables, fruits, and raw foods will enhance the positive impact on your cardiovascular well-being.

Mitigating the Cancer Risk

Vegetarianism has emerged as a potential safeguard against various types of cancer. These diets, low in saturated fat, high in fiber, and abundant in phytochemicals, have shown the ability to shield individuals from cancer risks.

Extensive studies conducted in England and Germany highlight that vegetarians possess a 40% lower chance of developing cancer compared to their meat-eating counterparts.

The Seventh-Day Adventists, largely adhering to a lacto-ovo vegetarian lifestyle, have been observed to have reduced cancer risks due to their avoidance of meat. In China, where vegetable consumption is prominent, reduced breast cancer rates have been documented. Conversely, Japanese women, who consume more meat, face an eight-fold increase in breast cancer risk.

Moreover, the consumption of meat and dairy products has been linked to other forms of cancer, including colon cancer, prostate cancer, and ovarian cancer.

Harvard studies involving thousands of women have revealed that regular meat consumption can increase the likelihood of colon cancer by 300%. High-fat diets common among meat eaters can lead to excess estrogen production, which, in turn, heightens the risk of breast cancer—particularly among premenopausal women.

Cambridge University has connected meat consumption to high levels of saturated fat, amplifying the risk of breast cancer. Dairy products, on the other hand, have been associated with an increased likelihood of ovarian cancer due to potential damage caused during the breakdown of lactose. In men, meat consumption has been linked to an elevated risk of prostate enlargement.

Boosting Digestive Wellness

Vegetarians often experience marked improvements in their digestive systems, creating a healthier and more natural environment for these vital organs. Our digestive systems were initially designed to process greater quantities of vegetable matter rather than meat.

Prehistoric diets revolved around fruits, vegetables, legumes, and nuts—the very staples that greatly benefit our digestive systems. Unfortunately, the Western diet has undergone drastic changes, embracing highly processed and refined foods. This shift has resulted in various health issues, ranging from heart disease to obesity.

When our bodies are not adequately nourished, and our digestive systems fail to function optimally, adaptations occur within our stomach and colon cells. Insufficient fiber intake often leads to complications such as constipation and hemorrhoids, conditions rarely encountered among those adhering to a vegetarian diet.

Shedding Excess Pounds

Weight management is a significant concern, particularly considering the prevailing obesity crisis. Have you ever encountered an overweight vegetarian? It's highly unlikely. In fact, most vegetarians maintain lean and healthy physiques.

Dieticians and nutritionists consistently recommend increasing vegetable intake while reducing meat consumption, particularly red meats and pork. Many individuals who revert to their previous diets find that the weight they lost rapidly returns.

Willpower alone cannot prevent weight gain resulting from high-fat, meat-based diets. By embracing a vegetarian lifestyle, you naturally provide your body with the nutrition it needs for sustainable energy, free from the need for excess fat storage.

You feel better and experience improved overall health. Traditional diets fail because they force us to resist foods we enjoy, ultimately tempting us to indulge. The key to successful vegetarianism lies in recognizing that you can thrive without meat and that you are focused on consuming healthier alternatives.

You'll be surprised to find yourself losing weight effortlessly simply by eliminating your primary source of unhealthy fats. Additionally, the negative health effects associated with high-fat diets vanish, thanks to your wholesome and natural food choices.

Renewed Kidney Health

Diets rich in animal proteins often lead to increased excretion of calcium, uric acid, and oxalates—common components of kidney stones. Individuals predisposed to kidney stones are advised by British researchers to adopt a vegetarian diet. The American Academy of Family Physicians has also confirmed that high animal protein consumption is a significant cause of kidney stones in the United States.

A vegetarian diet reduces the secretion of these substances, effectively reducing the risk of kidney stone formation.

Combating Osteoporosis

Just as vegetarianism lowers the risk of kidney stones, it also diminishes the chances of developing osteoporosis. Paradoxically, meat consumption can promote bone loss, as it contributes to calcium depletion within the body.

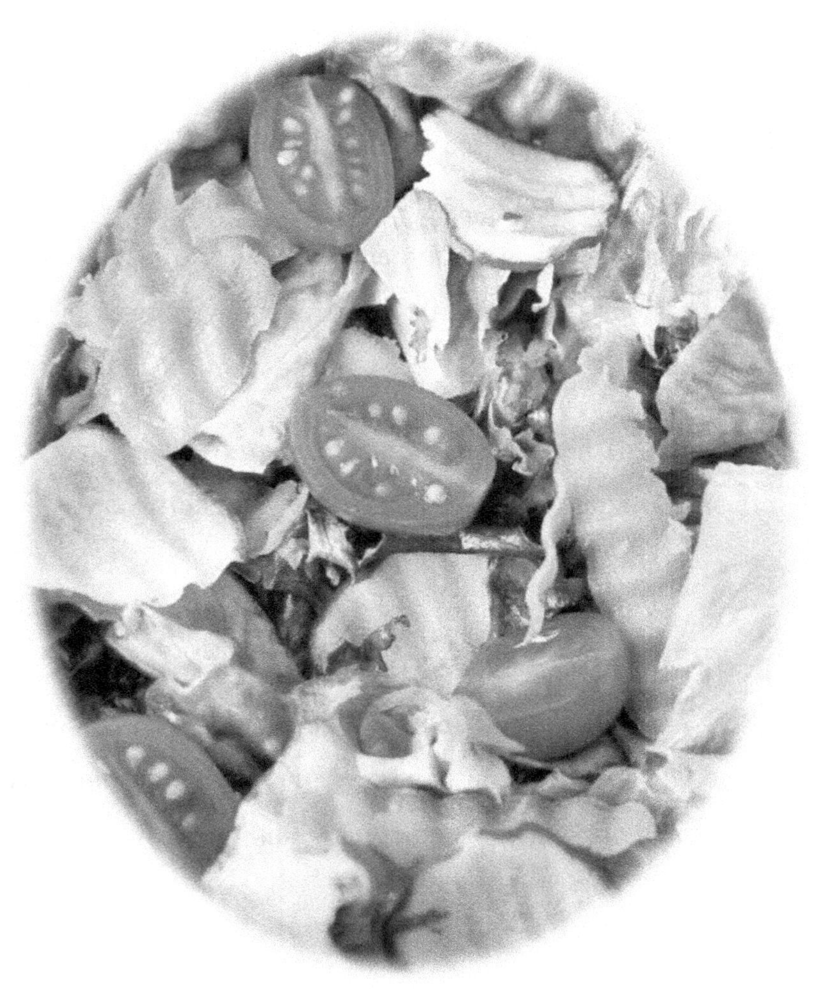

Embracing Vegetarianism as a Family

If you're contemplating a switch to a vegetarian diet, you'll likely want to share your newfound nutritional knowledge with your family. As a parent, ensuring that your family receives optimal nutrition and teaching them about the importance of healthy eating is crucial.

However, transitioning your entire family can be challenging, especially when children are enticed by fast-food restaurants and enticing snack commercials on television. After all, it's tough to compete with chicken nuggets and free toys!

Making gradual changes is key when transitioning your family's diet. It all begins at the grocery store. Instead of cookies, opt for apples, bananas, carrots, and other delicious snacks.

Swap white rice for nutritious brown rice, and steer clear of processed side dishes. Gradually reduce meat portions and increase the intake of vegetables and grains.

If you have young children, this switch is easier since you can introduce them to olives as tasty snacks and peaches as delightful desserts. They will grow to love these foods without even realizing the abundance of junk food options available. The real challenge comes when your children start making their own choices at school.

The idea is to make the transition gradually, ensuring it's easier for both you and your family. Many children are naturally empathetic, and when you explain that vegetarianism saves the lives of animals, they may willingly embrace it.

You're doing your children an enormous favor that will benefit them for a lifetime. Childhood obesity has reached epidemic levels in the US, and by teaching your children healthy eating habits now, you're setting them up for a lifetime of well-being.

You'll continue to use the same cooking supplies you already have, but you may need to dust off the blender and food processor if they aren't part of your regular routine.

Additionally, there are several new ingredients and foods that you'll be incorporating into your vegetarian diet, including:

Fruits & Vegetables

Grapes

Melon

Apples

Mushrooms

Avocado

Tomatoes

Oranges

Broccoli

Kiwi

Potatoes

Sweet Potatoes

Peppers

Cucumbers

Onions

Celery

Cherries

Plums

Carrots

Cabbage

Bananas

Egg Whites, Soy Milk & Dairy (unless you're giving them up)

Egg whites

Milk

Dairy milk

Soy milk

Dairy cheese

Soy cheese

Yogurt

Sauces & Oils

Olive oil

Rice vinegar

Toasted sesame oil

Groundnut oil

Tamari (Japanese soy sauce)

Hot chili oil

Seasonings

Black pepper

Curry powder

Dijon mustard

Fresh garlic

Fresh ginger

Sea salt

Herbs & Spices

Anise

Basil

Cayenne pepper

Chili powder

Cinnamon

Coriander

Cumin

Dill

Garlic powder

Nutmeg

Oregano

Paprika

Red chili flakes

Rosemary

Sage

Thyme

Noodles & Rice

Rice noodles

Soba noodles

Brown basmati rice

Nuts & Seeds

Almonds

Cashews

Peanuts

Sesame seeds

Sunflower seeds

Legumes

Black beans

Chickpeas

Lentils (red, green, and brown)

Split peas (yellow and green)

Kidney beans

Other

Coconut milk

Nutritional yeast

Pure maple syrup

Raw, unrefined sugar

Breakfast is an important meal that should never be skipped. Contrary to popular belief, consuming three proper meals a day can actually aid in weight loss. And breakfast doesn't have to be dull—it can be both delicious and nutritious.

Apple Cinnamon Granola

Ingredients:

4 cups oatmeal

1 cup wheat germ

1 tsp. ground cinnamon

A dash of nutmeg

½ cup finely chopped walnuts

½ cup honey

2 tbsp. sunflower oil

1 cup dried apples, finely chopped

½ cup raisins

Preheat the oven to 275 degrees Fahrenheit. In a large mixing bowl, combine oatmeal, wheat germ, cinnamon, nutmeg, and walnuts. In a separate bowl, mix honey and sunflower oil, then drizzle over the oat mixture.

Stir until evenly coated. Lightly oil a large baking sheet and spread the mixture onto it. Bake for 30 minutes, stirring every 10 minutes. Once the granola turns golden, remove from the oven and set aside to cool. Transfer the granola into jars and add dried apples and raisins. Store in a dry place. This recipe yields 6 cups.

Simple Crepes

Ingredients:

3 eggs

¾ cup + 2 tbsp. all-purpose flour

1 ½ cups milk

1 tbsp. granulated sugar

1 tbsp. vegetable oil

A pinch of salt

1 tsp. butter

Whipped cream (for filling)

Handfuls of strawberries, raspberries, and blueberries

Combine eggs, flour, milk, sugar, oil, and salt in a blender or food processor until smooth. Transfer the batter to a mixing bowl, cover, and refrigerate for at least 30 minutes.

In a non-stick skillet over medium-high heat, melt the butter. Pour ¼ cup of batter into the pan and swirl it to coat the entire bottom. Cook until the crepe lightly browns on one side, then flip and cook the other side until lightly browned.

Transfer to plates and fill with whipped cream and a handful of mixed berries. Fold the sides gently to form a cylinder. This recipe yields 8 to 12 crepes.

Vegetable Omelet

Ingredients:

2 eggs

3 tbsp. milk

A big pinch of salt

A big pinch of black pepper

1 tbsp. butter

¼ cup green bell pepper

¼ cup red bell pepper

¼ cup onion

Grated cheese (optional)

In a medium-sized mixing bowl, beat eggs, salt, pepper, green and red peppers, and onion with a fork. Do not overmix. Melt butter in a 7 to 8-inch pan over medium-high heat, ensuring the butter covers the base of the pan. Once the foam subsides, pour in the egg mixture.

Tilt the pan to ensure the egg covers the entire base. Let the eggs set for 45 seconds before flipping. Cook the other side for the same duration. Transfer to a plate and sprinkle with grated cheese if desired.

Smoothies

Smoothies are not only healthy but also delicious. They can be enjoyed as snacks or as part of your brunch.

Breakfast Smoothies

Ingredients:

1 ½ cups plain fat-free yogurt

3 to 4 bananas

3 cups strawberries (stems removed and roughly chopped)

¼ cup soy milk

2 tbsp. honey

1 cup ice

Blend the ingredients one at a time in a blender and serve.

Banana and Yogurt Smoothie

Ingredients:

1 ripe banana, thinly sliced

1 cup low-fat plain or vanilla yogurt

¾ cup skim milk

Set aside a few banana slices for garnish. In a blender, combine the remaining banana slices, yogurt, and milk. Blend until smooth. Pour into glasses, garnish with banana slices, and sprinkle with cinnamon.

Mango Smoothie

Ingredients:

1 mango, peeled and chopped

1 banana, peeled

3 tbsp. yogurt

1 tsp. honey

½ tsp. cinnamon

4 ice cubes

Add the ingredients to a blender one at a time and puree until smooth.

Pear Smoothie

Ingredients:

3 pears

½ inch fresh ginger

3 tbsp. fresh yogurt

½ tsp. cinnamon

4 ice cubes

Juice the pears, ginger, and cinnamon together. Transfer to a blender and add yogurt and ice. Blend until smooth.

Appetizers & Side Dishes

These dishes make excellent sides to a healthy meal or delightful appetizers. They can even be enjoyed as snacks!

Special Tomato Bruschetta

Ingredients:

4 bread rolls

4 garlic cloves

2 tbsp. butter

1 tbsp. chopped basil

4 large tomatoes

1 tbsp. tomato paste

8 black olives, pitted and halved

1 ¾ ounce mozzarella cheese, sliced

Salt and pepper to taste

1 tbsp. olive oil

2 tsp. lemon juice or balsamic vinegar

1 tsp. clear honey

Basil leaves for garnish

Place the rolls on a cutting board and slice each in half. Toast the rolls in a toaster oven or oven until they become brown and crisp. Preheat the oven to 300 degrees Fahrenheit. In a small mixing bowl, combine butter, garlic, and chopped basil. Once the rolls are toasted, spread the garlic mixture onto each half.

Place the tomatoes in boiling water, make a small cross-shaped cut at the base of each tomato, and then put them in the boiling water. Once the tomatoes soften, remove them and peel away the skin. Chop the flesh into small squares. In a mixing bowl, blend the diced tomatoes, tomato paste, and olives. Spoon the mixture onto the rolls.

In a separate bowl, mix olive oil, lemon juice or balsamic vinegar, and honey. Drizzle the mixture over the tomato-covered rolls and place mozzarella slices on top. Sprinkle with salt and pepper. Place the rolls on a baking sheet and bake until the cheese melts (approximately 2 minutes). Transfer the rolls to a platter or tray, garnish with basil leaves, and serve.

Ingredients for Spring Rolls:

¾ cup broken rice vermicelli noodles

6 fresh shiitake mushrooms

½ cup slivered carrots

1 cup sliced bok choy

1 cup slivered green onions

2 tbsp. chopped coriander

Salt and ground pepper to taste

2 tbsp. soy sauce

½ tsp. granulated sugar

1 tsp. sesame oil

Eight 8-inch square spring roll skins

3 tbsp. all-purpose flour

¼ cup water

4 cups vegetable oil

Ingredients for Salad:

1 cup slivered daikon radish

1 cup slivered carrots

4 slivered green onions

½ cup slivered red onion

1 cup slivered cucumber (squeeze out excess juice)

Ingredients for Dressing:

2 tbsp. seasoned rice vinegar

1 tbsp. soy sauce

½ tsp. sesame oil

Soak the rice vermicelli noodles and shiitake mushrooms in separate bowls of hot water. Cover the bowls and let them soak for 20 minutes. Drain and transfer them to a colander.

Thinly slice the mushrooms, removing and discarding the stems. In a large bowl, combine the noodles, mushrooms, carrots, bok choy, green onions, coriander, salt, pepper, soy sauce, sugar, and sesame oil. Mix well and set aside.

Gently separate the spring roll skins and place them on a clean, flat surface. Place ¼ cup of the noodle and vegetable mixture on the upper third of each skin. Roll once, fold in the two ends, and continue rolling to form a cylinder.

In a small bowl, whisk together flour and water to form a paste. Use a small pastry brush to seal the edges of the spring rolls with the paste. Repeat for all rolls.

In a wok, heat vegetable oil over medium-high heat. Fry the spring rolls in batches until they turn golden brown. Transfer them to a rack lined with paper towels to drain excess oil.

To make the salad, combine daikon radish, carrots, green onions, red onion, and cucumber in a bowl. In a separate bowl, whisk together seasoned rice vinegar, soy sauce, and sesame oil. Toss the dressing with the salad ingredients.\

Slice each spring roll in half diagonally and serve with the salad on the side.

Pita Pizza

Ingredients:

¼ tsp. olive oil

½ small onion, diced

1 clove garlic, minced

¼ tsp. dried oregano

¼ tsp. dried basil

¼ tsp. crushed red pepper flakes

1 bay leaf

½ cup canned whole peeled tomatoes, roughly chopped

½ cup tomato paste

2 whole wheat pita breads

½ yellow bell pepper, cut into thin strips

1/8 cup chopped baby spinach

½ cup grated mozzarella cheese

Fresh basil for garnish

Preheat

CONCLUSION

Throughout this guide, we've explored the numerous benefits of vegetarianism, from improving your overall well-being to reducing environmental impact. By choosing plant-based foods, you're not only nourishing your body but also making a positive difference in the world.

Transitioning to a vegetarian diet may seem challenging at first, especially when faced with the temptations of fast food and convenience snacks. However, armed with the knowledge and practical tips provided in this guide, you have the power to make sustainable choices for yourself and your family.

By gradually incorporating delicious fruits, vegetables, legumes, and grains into your meals, you'll discover a whole new world of flavors and textures.

Moreover, your journey towards vegetarianism can extend beyond the dinner table. With the abundance of ethical and eco-friendly products available today, you can make conscious choices when it comes to clothing, personal care items, and household products. By embracing a holistic approach to vegetarianism, you're aligning your values with your actions, creating a positive ripple effect in the world around you.

Remember, embracing vegetarianism is not about sacrifice or deprivation; it's about embracing a lifestyle filled with vibrant flavors, improved health, and a greater sense of connection with the planet.

As you embark on this journey, surround yourself with like-minded individuals, join vegetarian communities, and continue to educate yourself about the benefits of plant-based living.

So, go forth with confidence, armed with the knowledge and inspiration to live a greener, more compassionate life. Embrace the power of vegetarianism, and let it guide you towards a brighter, healthier, and more sustainable future for yourself and generations to come.

Together, we can make a meaningful difference and create a world where the choice to embrace vegetarianism is not only a personal one but a collective responsibility for the well-being of our planet.

www.ingramcontent.com/pod-product-compliance
Lightning Source LLC
Chambersburg PA
CBHW080240260726
48658CB00008B/3181